ABOUT THE AUTHOR

Scott J Connor ©

I0505386

Table of Contents

HOMEMADE MEDICAL FACE MASK

THE SIMPLEST STEP BY STEP

GUIDE TO CREATE A HOMEMADE

FACE MASK FOR VIRUS

PROTECTION.

*PROTECT YOURSELF AND YOUR FAMILY
FROM VIRUSES AND INFECTIONS USING
FACE MASK AND HAND SANITIZER*

Scott J Connor

CHAPTER 1:

VIRUS PROTECTION

Germs exist everywhere we go. Germs, viruses are tiny organisms (microbes) that can be found in water, air, the food we eat, and on just about every surface, your body is not excluded from the list.

Many of the germs do you no good. The immune system protects you against infectious agents. Some germs are hard enemies, though, because they continuously mutate to destroy the immune system's defenses. Knowing how germs work will increase the chances of avoiding infection.

What is the safest way? Preventing infection, such as, will avoid infections, regularly wash your hands, avoid physical contact with sick people, scrub regularly touched surfaces, avoid contaminated food and water, vaccinate, and take necessary medicines, and most importantly, using face masks.

When germs come into the body, they're planning to live for a while. The host gets all their energy from these germs. They can damage healthy cells or kill them. They can create proteins known as toxins as they eat their nutrients and energy, which will aid the germ in its quest to kill them.

Germs also stimulate the immune system, the network of cells, tissues and organs that function to defend the body together. Our immune system sends white blood cells, antibodies, and other chemicals into the body to destroy invading germs.

Processes of germs, toxins, and the immune system may cause alarming symptoms of a cold or flu-like infection, such as the runny nose, sneezing, cough, and diarrhea. They may also cause high fever, higher heart rate, low blood pressure, an inflammatory body response, and even life-threatening disease.

Virus Protection Mask

Viruses like this can work in many ways. Viruses originally are meant to be unable to survive outside bodily fluids. This means that if they are just on their own, they would not survive. However, when viruses are in bodily fluids and liquids such as saliva, sweat, blood, and other body fluids, they can be transferred from the infected person to someone not yet infected. This is the reason why the virus, Human Immunodeficiency Virus (HIV) is very deadly. It exists in the blood of infected individuals and moves on to another individual when there is some sort of contact with such blood. Viruses that affect the respiratory system also act like that. These viruses have to exist in the saliva, or nasal fluid droplets of an infected individual. Hence, they move from one person to another when such person sneezes or coughs. These drops may also be spread by rubbing your eyes and nose and then rubbing another person or surface. If anyone comes into contact with these infectious droplets, either in the air or by touching a droplet-containing surface, they can get sick too.

Any kind of masks will be good because they cover your nose and mouth, so they don't touch them but keep your eyes open so you can contact and spread the virus this way.

Masks are a tool for stopping the disease from spreading. These masks have been given different names, from dental masks, isolation masks, medical protective masks, surgical masks and so on. They are called these names primarily because of the job they do, they protect your face, especially the mouth and nose. The way they are designed, you can either wear them and hang the hooks on your ears or tie the ribbons at the back of your head.

The face masks help to reduce germ spread. They can disperse tiny droplets into the air when an infected individual speaks, coughs, or sneezes that can affect others. A face mask can minimize the number of germs produced by the user when someone is sick and protect other people from the disease. Often, a face mask protects the wearer's nose and mouth from body fluid splashes or sprays.

If you have a cough or sneeze (with or without fever), wear a face mask, and plan to be with other people. The mask protects you from illness. Unique guidelines apply when people have to wear face masks in health-care environments.

Face Mask Types That Exist Currently

These are the currently available face mask types that can be used in reducing the spread of germs or preventing the penetration of viruses.

Homemade Masks

To maintain a strategic distance from utilizers from spreading to individuals, it is currently suggested that everybody wear face covers of texture, for instance. The face veils are carefully assembled. This counsel supplements current social removing exercises and great cleanliness.

Proposals include: Wear fabric face covers openly puts, particularly in territories with generous transmission at the network level, for example, grocery stores and drug stores. Try not to put texture veils on kids under two years old, individuals with respiratory issues, oblivious individuals, or other people who cannot discard the cover. Wear fabric veils rather than careful covers or N95 respirators, as these fundamental things must be held for crisis work force and other emergency treatment drugs. Wellbeing experts should show incredible alert when utilizing face covers made without anyone else.

Benefits Of Homemade Face Masks

- Homemade face masks can be made from common household products, so supply is limitless.

- This may reduce the risk of people spreading the virus by talking, coughing, or sneezing without symptoms.
- Hats are better than not wearing a mask and provide some protection, particularly when it's difficult to maintain social distancing.

Homemade Face Masks Risks

- This can convey a false sense of trust. Albeit custom made face covers give some security, they furnish substantially less assurance contrasted and careful covers or respirators. Hand crafted covers can be as compelling as careful veils and as incredible as N95 covers up to a minimum of 50 times less.
- They don't substitute or minimize the need for other protections. Proper grooming and social distancing activities are also the best ways to cover yourself.

Surgical Masks

Surgical masks are flexible, removable masks that cover the chin, nose, and ears. Typically, you are used to: Cover the consumer with large particles from aerosols, splashes, and drops.

Forestalling the way in which these contagious diseases are dispersed from the patient to other Surgical veils can contrast in size. All things considered, with folds or wrinkles, the veil itself is generally level and rectangular. The surface of the mask comprises a strip of metal that can be molded around the nose.

When wearing it, flexible groups or tight, straight ties hold a careful veil set up. This can be mounted or tied behind the head.

N95 Respirator

An N95 fan is a face mask attached to it. This fan can likewise evacuate 95 percent of exceptionally little particles notwithstanding sprinkles, splashes, and large beads. This includes Bacteria and Viruses.

The fan itself is normally circular or oval and is designed to seal your face tightly. The bands of rubber hold it tightly against your nose. Some forms may have an attachment called an exhalation valve that can help breathe, and heat and moisture accumulate.

N95 Breathers aren't one size fits all. Until utilized, they ought to be tried for fit to guarantee that a legitimate seal is framed. Unless the mask doesn't successfully cover your face, you won't get enough protection.

Users of N95 respirators will carry out a leak test any time they wear it after the fittest. It is also important to note that in certain groups, hermetic sealing is not achievable. This includes those with facial hair and babies.

Simple mouth and nose protection were traditionally used almost exclusively in operating rooms, a mask made of a relatively thin paper fleece bound with ribbons behind the ear.

This mouthguard is mainly used by doctors and assistants to keep their patients from being contaminated on the operating table with germs and pathogens. For instance, if the mask wearer coughs or sneezes, most drops are caught in the mask from the mouth and throat.

Over the long term, though, this only works if the mask is periodically changed and hygienically and properly disposed of. Doctors will adjust the mask at least every two hours during surgery. On the other hand, if there is the frequent use of such a mask, it easily loses its effectiveness.

CHAPTER 2

Masks that use replaceable filters

1. Points of interest

As a very important matter, you ought to always wash your mask immediately it gets dirty. The cover can be washed day by day if you want or as regularly as possible. It will unmistakably negatively affect the mask on the off chance that you wash it more consistently than not. Hence, in any event it looks clean and is liberated from particles which you in any case may take in.

Second, you have the likelihood to check the channel routinely. You can genuinely perceive how much air contamination there is. Much more in this way, you get a smart thought how soon you need to change the channel. When the outside of the channel is dim or dark, you ought to quickly supplant it. The channel proficiency is no more. Furthermore, the dim or dark issue are the fine particles that you in any case would breath if you don't wear a face or nose mask. It is a genuine eye opener, I let you know, particularly the first time when you see it.

2. Disadvantages

All things considered, to take the most exceedingly awful first: the issue is that replaceable channels by and large don't cover the full region of the mask. However, to counter that contention, you have to see how the particles enter your body. It is obviously that it is mostly imperative to cover the zone around your nose and mouth. While breathing, this is the place and how the particles get to you and into your body. Therefore, so far you can keep the nose and mouth parts of your face (and more clearly) secured with a channel, you have got enough protection.

Masks that do not use replaceable filters

1. Preferences

The Number 1 and just preferred position of masks without replaceable channels is that the channel covers the entire zone of the mask. However, given that it's for the most part imperative to cover the zone where you breath in, it doesn't generally make a difference whether it is covering the entire mask or not. As referenced over, the fine particles just enter your body through your mouse or nose. In that sense, you are wealthy simply getting a mask which has a replaceable filter.

2. Hindrances

The serious issue with non-replaceable channels/ filters is that you can't check in what condition your filter is. Given, there are some masks that can give you an application with which you can verify how efficient it is or not. Therefore, what amount does that help, if you need to discard the entire cover and purchase another one at any rate? Moreover, these veils are likewise celebrated for their extravagance status and will cost you oodles of cash (30-40 USD per cover). Pose yourself this inquiry: would you say you will spend around 30-40 USD each 1-2 months?

Additionally, the masks which have an in-manufactured channel are not launderable, at any rate not so much. You can take a freely wet fabric and attempt to clear off the outside of the mask. Within the cover will be hard to wash. What's more, the most concerning issue is that the filter can't

11

be expelled before washing and henceforth making it wet would make your filter ineffectual.

How much protection does the mask provide?

The mask holder can shield himself from gout and smear infections, but just to a small degree. While the virus usually enters the body through the mouth or eyes, the hands play the most important role in the transportation of the virus, if there are no open wounds.

You will probably choose glasses too if you want a mask. Although surgical masks are less effective in keeping the virus away, they only act as a constant reminder that your hands should not touch your nose when itchy. Not rubbing your eyes, either.

Half Masks Offer Better Protection

Including surgical masks that are more like multilayer disposable kitchen towels, there are half masks with a real filter effect as well. Many who operate in dusty or aerosolized conditions are better known for these. They are available as disposable masks, typically made of heavily pressed cellulose with a filter feature and exhalation valve, or as plastic masks in which an appropriate filter is installed afterward.

Some types of masks in the European Union are classified into three groups of FFP (filter front) safety. Although FFP1 security masks are better still than surgical masks, they do not provide the necessary virus protection. For example, they are intended for carpenters having a vacuum extraction system operating on a bandsaw. Workers will take them to get the thickest dust the vacuum cleaner can't find. Or they can be placed on by a mason before mixing cement with a trowel and spinning a small powder.

Even FFP-3 type masks effectively protect the user against droplet, protein molecules, viruses, bacteria, fungi, and spores aerosols and even highly dangerous dust such as asbestos fibers.

Thanks to their nature, these high-quality filter masks, unlike basic surgical masks, can shield the wearer from infection. In other words, with a highly infectious agent such as measles or tuberculosis.

But here, too, security works only if many other preventive measures are taken simultaneously: strict hygiene when putting on a mask, safety glasses, gloves, and a plastic apron or, generally, careful disposal of potentially disposable items. Additionally, the environment must always be regularly disinfected.

For example, these masks, along with all other protective clothing, are used in quarantine stations, where infected patients are taken care of. With great effort, medical personnel must put on and take off all protective equipment, including protective mask.

This commitment will be somewhat unnecessary while traveling on public transport or operating on changing offices with a mouse, which are among the worst germs.

CHAPTER 3

HOW TO MAKE THE MOST EFFECTIVE VIRUS PROTECTION FACE MASK

If you are around other men, there is still anxiety about the spread of germs. For example, if you ride every day to and from work on a crowded subway or other public transportation, you may be worried that the person sitting next to you will be noticed. You will effectively remove some of the contaminants in the air by using a surgical mask or certain forms of respirators (including certain viruses) that could otherwise touch you. Having that in mind, wearing a surgical mask will provide you with additional security and health, particularly if you spend time regularly in large crowds.

It's important to note that using a surgical mask (also widely referred to as a mouth mask) does not necessarily protect you against some viruses (or other viruses in the air) capture. Also, N95 masks, one of the most effective face masks available, can block only around 95 percent of small particles when used correctly (hence the filtration efficiency name

N95). Of the seven types of particulate filter respirators, the N95 respirator is the most common. This drug filters at least 95% of airborne particulate matter or N95 particulate matter, but is not oil resistant.

You want your physical weaknesses to understand too. Surgical masks can reduce the flow of air, which can be a concern for people with breathing issues (such as asthma).

However, it will be ideal if you can make use of a homemade virus protection mask. They are easy to make, and affordable, easy to breathe with.

Here Is A Practical Guide On How To Make A Face Mask At Home-Sew Method

Materials needed:

- One piece of cloth sized 8" x 14". Till you get used to the tutorial, I would suggest a non-directional print.
- Two small pieces of 1/4" width elastic, about 6 1/2" long.
- Two strips of cloth measuring 1.75" (1 3/4") x 6.
- Pins
- Fabric marking tool.
- Sewing machine, threaded.

- Scissors

1. Fold the central piece of fabric together in half, on the right side. Sew around the edge of the 8-inch length, using a seam allowance of 1/4 inch.

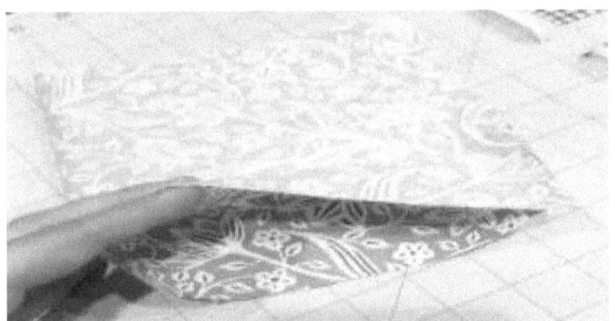

2. Turn the blueprint of this cylinder back to front, so the texture's correct side is presently outside. Push this level and hold the crease to one finish of the level pipeline.

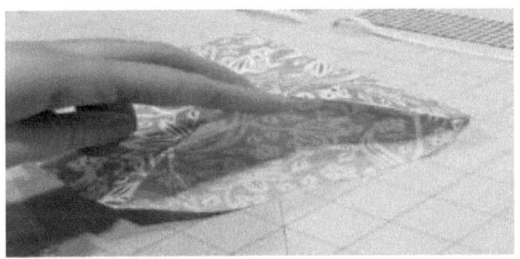

3. Spot the container of texture with the goal that the crude edges are both sides, and the creased end is at the bottom. Utilizing a measuring tape or a rule, get the dimensions needed and imprint a line above half distance

from the base edge. Make a different line 1 inch over this line, Try, not to utilize a pencil as you find in the image, utilize a texture pen, or texture chalk. I utilized a pencil for delineation purposes.

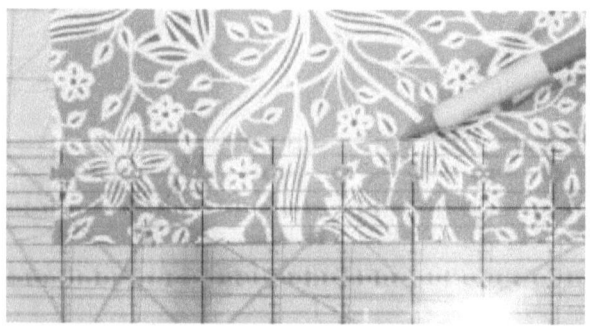

4.   Overlap the creased edge up (or , as shown in this image, down), making the wrinkle on the principal line you simply checked. You ought to have half inch edge.

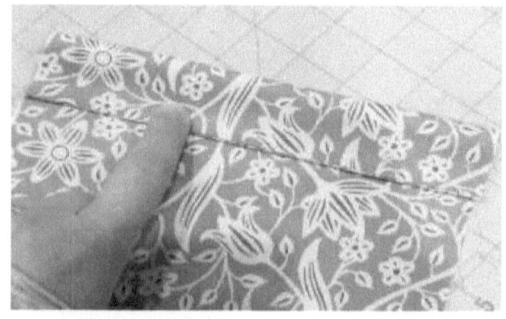

5.   Flip the cylinder piece over. Match the wrinkle edge to the next line that you had made before. Press. The wrinkle

that you have just made will be half inch down. Nail the crease down on every crude edge end.

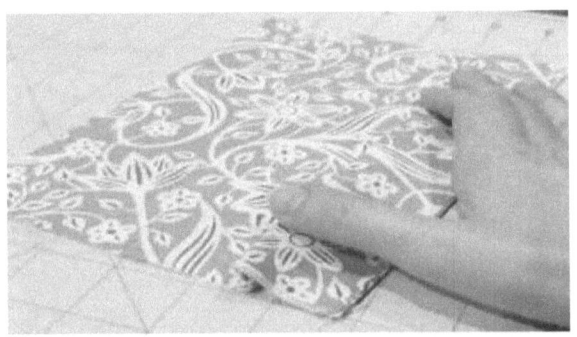

6.   Presently mark a different line few centimeters over the last line that you made (or 3 crawls over the crease edge).

Utilizing the first lines as your guide, rehash the means that you took when making the principal crease.

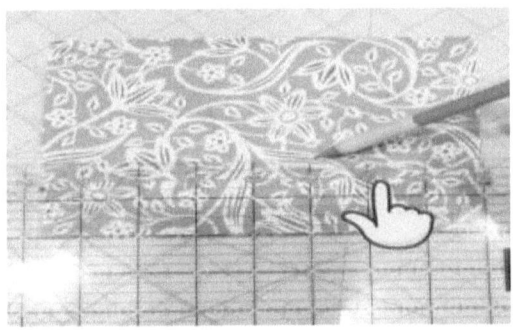

7.   You should presently see two creases, every one being half inch down. Rehash the means you used in making

the subsequent wrinkle so you come out with three creases all out.

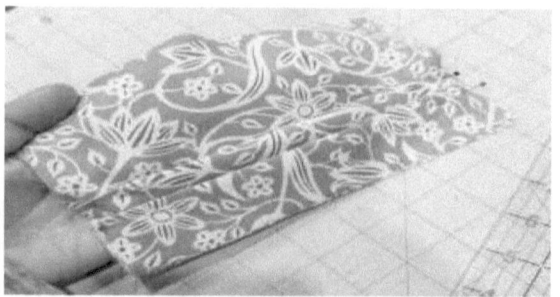

This is how the main piece should be looking like currently.

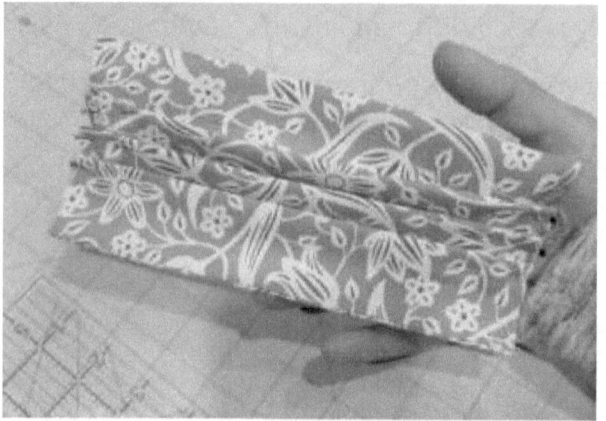

Using a one eight inch allowance for the seam, get the raw edges basted.

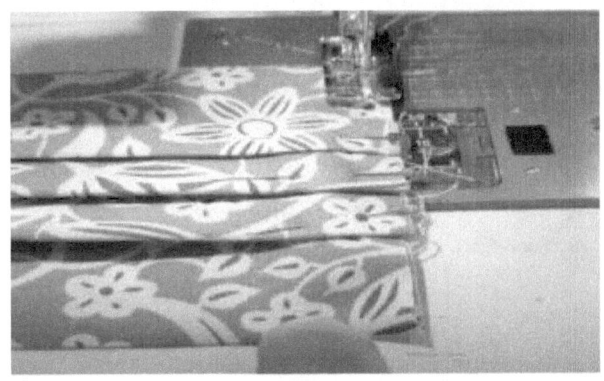

Do this step again to allow both edges to be basted.

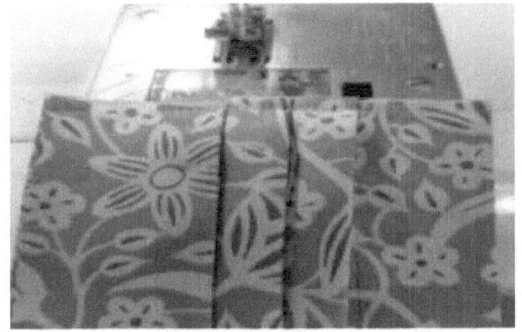

8.   Pin one versatile piece to the crude edge, making a point not to turn it before season sewing it to the edge at the two finishes. I set mine 1/8" from the top and base edge of the fundamental creased piece. Season flexible set up 1/8" inch from the crude edge. Rehash to append the staying flexible piece to the next crude edge.

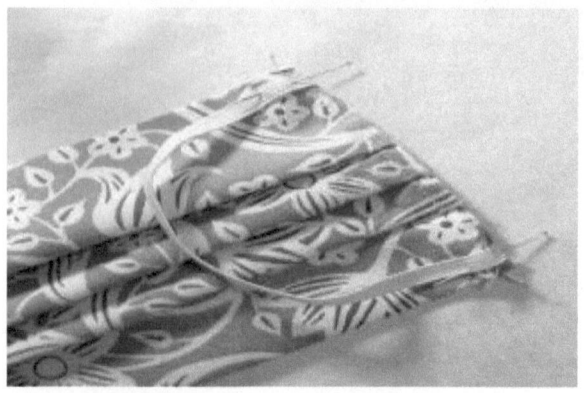

Your pleated piece should look like the picture below by now

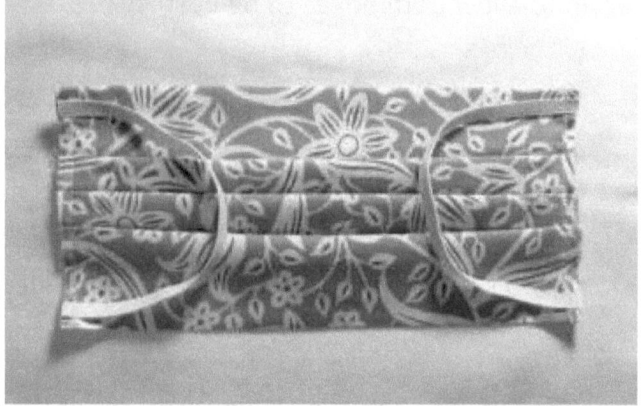

Fold each accent strip of fabric lengthwise in half, matching raw edges

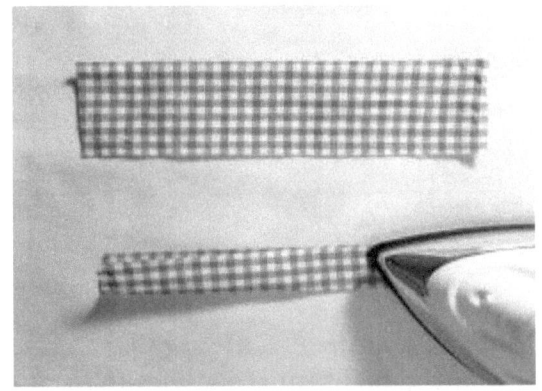

9.   Place the strip on top of the elastic. Make sure the raw edge is facing outward, and the creased edge is facing the main body of the pleated piece. It will be a little longer on the top and bottom, and that is okay, as we are going to fold some of that to the back.

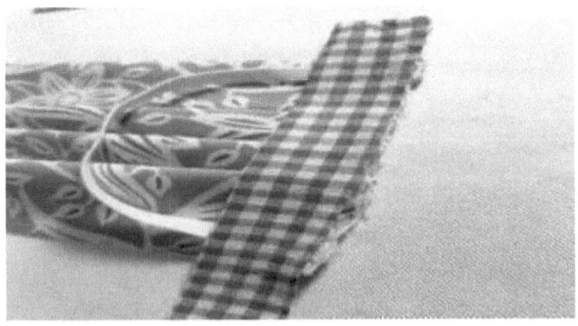

Tuck in about half inch of the mask's top edge to the mask's back.

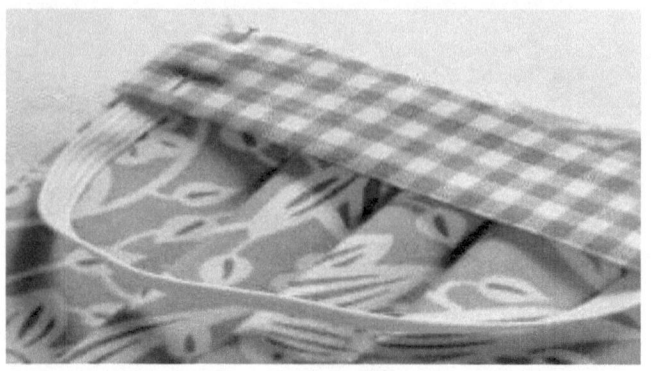

Trim the opposite finish of the highlight strip, with the goal that it is around 1/2" longer than the base edge of the principle creased piece.

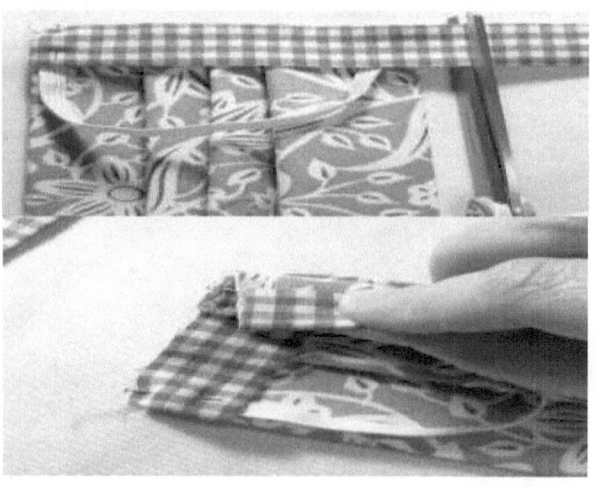

Crease the base of the complement texture cloth to the back, similarly as you had earlier done with the other surface.

Pin the two finishes set up.

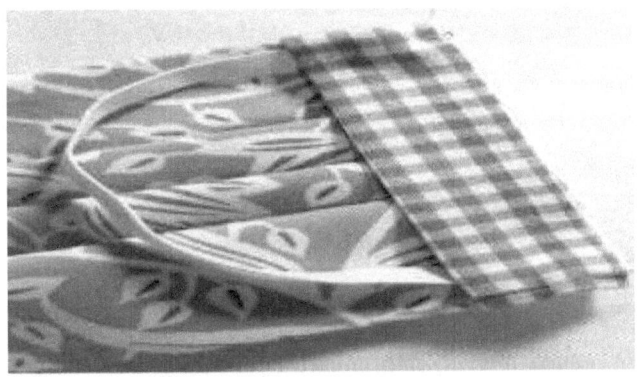

Utilizing a quarter inch crease space, fasten the whole of the edge, making a point to backstitch toward the start and end.

Open the texture strip crease by turning it outwards from the fundamental creased piece, at that point press.

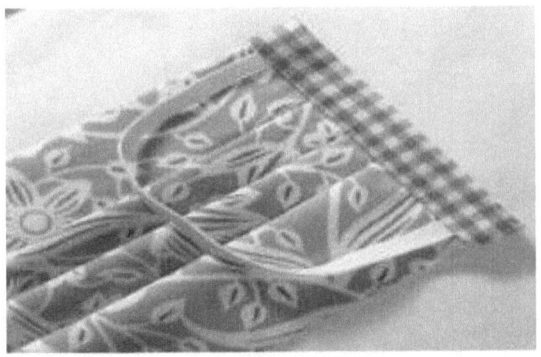

This is how the mask should be looking like when you put it to its other side.

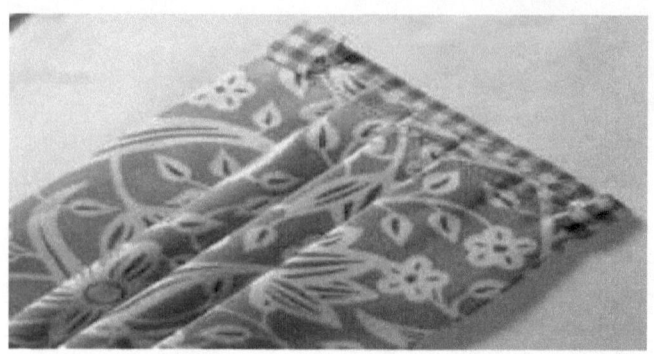

crease the ENTIRE inflection piece down toward the principle creased piece, encasing the crude crease. You will presently observe the complement piece on this site, yet not in any way on the other side. Pin edge down.

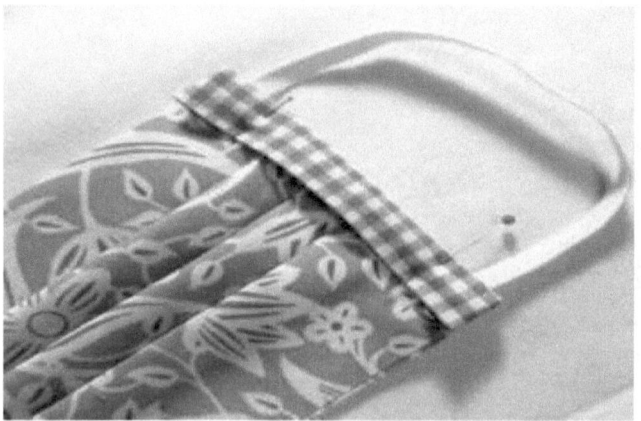

On the off chance that you have some decent tailoring skills, you can go ahead to remove the other end for the straight end. In the event that you are languid, similar to me, you can use the pedal of the machine and keep at it all through the sewing. Join this complement strip to the primary body of the cover, sewing along the edge, so that it makes a point to backstitch toward the start and end.

This progression isn't important. It just gives it a pleasant completed look and assists with giving that versatile some additional strength. Fasten down the edge of the cover near the flexible side.

The front side and back of it should look like;

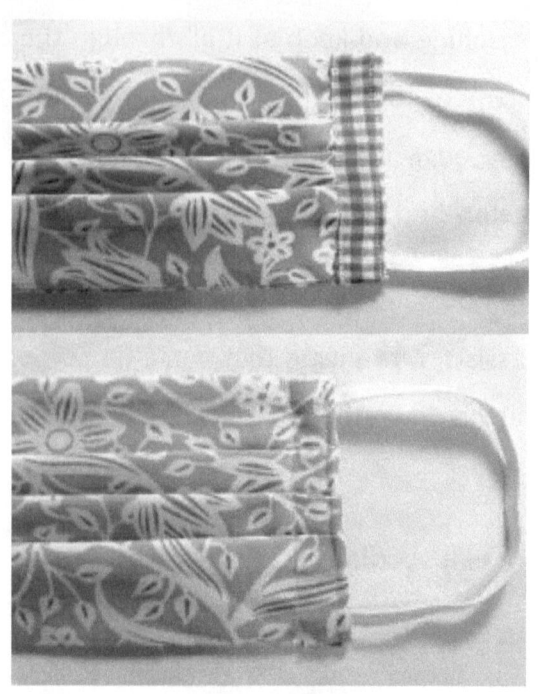

Now, you should have a 4 by 7 inch mask that you can use more than once after washing.

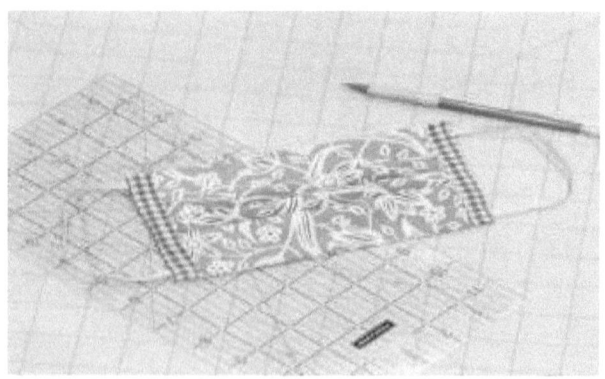

NO-SEW METHOD

Quick Cut T-Shirt Face Covering (No Sew Method)

Materials

- Scissors or Blade
- A T-shirt

1.

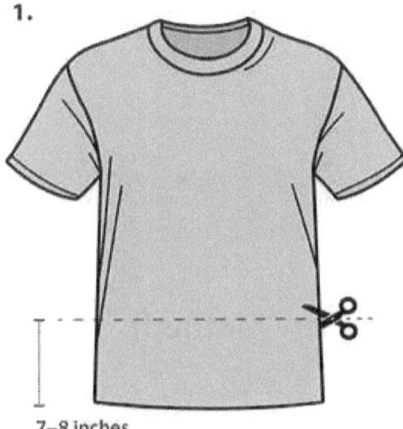

7–8 inches

2.

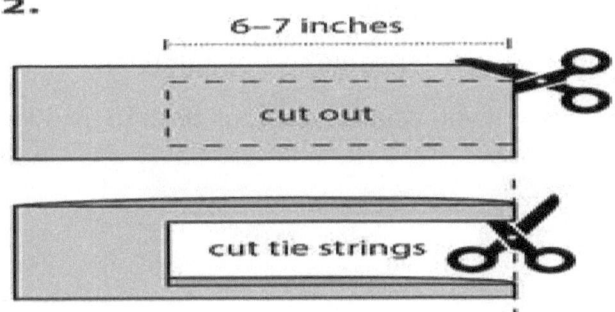

6–7 inches

cut out

cut tie strings

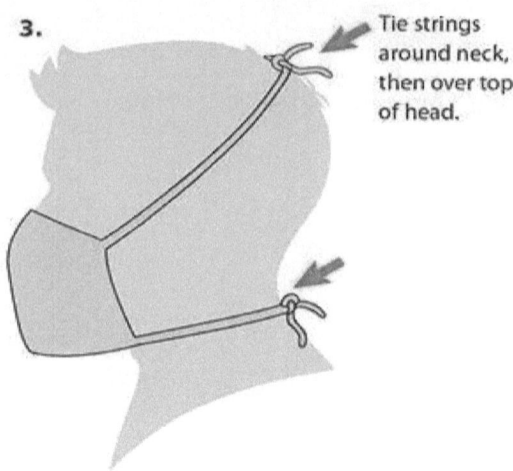

3. Tie strings around neck, then over top of head.

CHAPTER 4

Bandana Face Covering (No Sew Method)

Materials

- Bandana (or any square cotton cloth size 20" x20")
- Rubber bands (or some sort of hair ties)
- Scissors (if you want to cut your cloth to use) **Tutorial**

1.

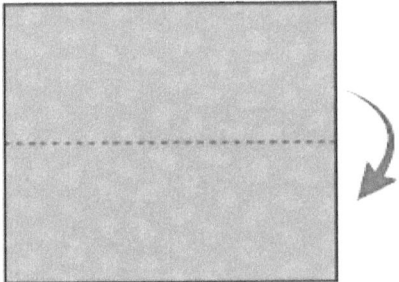

Fold bandana in half.

2.

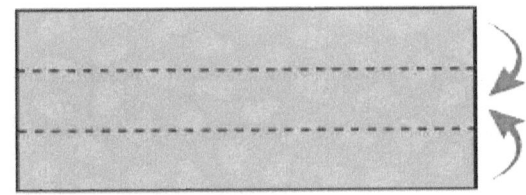

Fold top down. Fold bottom up.

3.

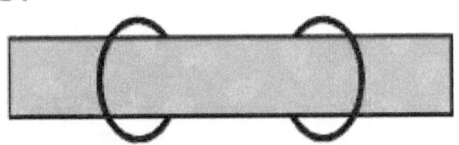

Place rubber bands or hair ties
about 6 inches apart.

4.

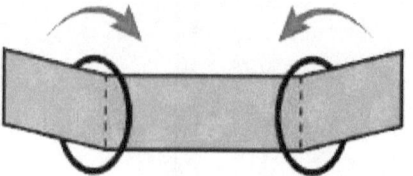

Fold side to the middle and tuck.

5.

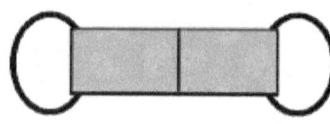

6.

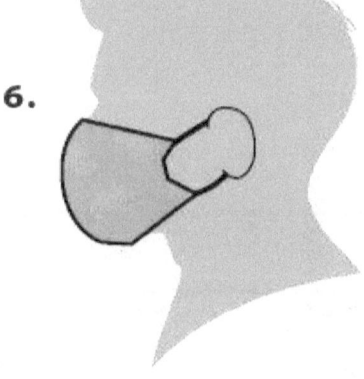

The Best Material To Use For Making Homemade Face Masks

Many people would have to settle for what some scientists have called "the last resort": the DIY mask with the goggles.

The data indicate that the viruses are caught effectively by homemade and DIY masks. But if you're forced to make our cover, what better material to make a cover?

Researchers at the University of Cambridge examined various types of home materials for homemade masks. They fired the bacteria, Bacillus atrophaeus, (0.93-1.25 microns) and MS bacteriophage virus (0.023 microns) into various household materials to test the effectiveness.

They looked for what percentage can be absorbed by the materials and compared to the most popular surgical mask.

The surgical mask performed best, not surprisingly, and contained 97 percent of the 1-micron bacteria. However, at least 50 percent of the particles were filtered by each material. The best results were the vacuum cleaner bag which held 95%, the kitchen cloth ("kitchen cloth" in Great

Britain! 83%), the shirt fabric made of the cotton blend (74%), and the shirt made 100% cotton (69%).

Homemade masks vs. Viruses

The previous study used one micron-sized bacteria, but the coronavirus is just 0.1 micron, ten times smaller. Can homemade masks trap particles smaller than the virus? The scientists measured 0.02-micron bacteriophage particles of MS2 (5 times smaller than coronavirus) to answer that question.

Homemade masks produced 7 percent fewer virus particles on average than larger particles of bacteria. All household products, however, could catch 50 percent or more of the virus particles (except 49 percent of the scarf).

The double layers weren't helping much in general. The two-layer pillowcase contained 1 percent more particles, and only 2 percent more particles were absorbed by the two-layer shirt. The additional layer of tea towels, however, improved efficiency by 14 percent. This boost made both the dishcloth and the surgical mask as effective.

In terms of results, the best materials have been the dishcloth and the vacuum cleaner bag. The researchers did not say one material was better than the other in making DIY masks, however:

Instead, they concluded that DIY masks made with the right fabrics from a pillowcase and 100 percent cotton Tshirt are the best. Why? Because breathability is the key.

How easily you can breathe through the mask influences comfort. And comfort doesn't just mean luxury. Comfort influences how long you are permitted to wear your mask.

Fortunately, the researchers measured the pressure drop in each type of tissue, in addition to the particle efficacy. This gives us a clear example of the simplicity of breathing in any material.

Though most of the particles were trapped in the dishcloth and vacuum bag, they were also the most difficult to breath through. The dishcloth was more than twice as difficult to breathe with two layers, as was the surgical mask. By comparison, it was easier to breathe the pillowcase, T-shirt, scarf, and linen than the surgical mask.

CHAPTER 5

HOW TO WEAR PROPERLY FACE MASKS TO PREVENT VIRUS

It was recommended that Americans can use them voluntarily to prevent the spread of viruses, masks have become a common sight recently. Nevertheless, several people abuse the masks, which can impact how well they protect you and others against viruses.

The face masks have to fit snugly against the side of a person's face, according to the CDC. The WHO says there should be no holes between the face and mask covering the whole mouth and nose.

Health experts emphasize that people need to not have some false sense of protection owing to the fact that they are wearing a mask. The mask is not a shield. It is more precautionary than protective. The CDC also does not allow the use of surgical masks or N95s for emergency treatment and other front-line staff.

Here are some do's and don'ts for wearing a mask.

Do's

1. Wash your hands thoroughly before you wear your mask

The mask comes in near touch with your nose and ears. Please make sure to use clean hands before putting on. Ensure you wash your hands and do so thoroughly. This should be for a minimum of 20 seconds, with water and detergent. If you don't have access to water and soap, a hand sanitizer can also be used.

2. Ensure the mask is properly worn, such that it covers the nose and mouth.

When you wear a mask, you impede the distribution of water droplets in the air. The CDC revised its wearing masks guidelines as research found that people with coronaviruses were able to pass the disease on to others until they had symptoms or had no symptoms. Multilayer masks often help filter droplets out before they reach the face, although cloth masks are less successful than N95 respirators.

It should be as close to the face as possible and cover the mouth and nose to the nose bridge for the mask to be most effective.

3.   Utilize the ear loops while removing the mask

Utilize the mask's ear loops when removing the mask so as not to touch it. Discard it in a shut container, and quickly wash your face. Seek not to reach the mask front, which is capable of holding germs.

4.   Wash your cloth masks

"Routinely washing cloth masks depends on the level of use." This does not offer any detail about how much you can wash a mask, but the company claims a washing machine is enough to clean a cloth mask.

5.   Only wear your mask when necessary

Wearing a handmade mask won't stop you immediately from getting viruses attacks. For a homemade mask, you will be unable to create a barrier around your face just like the way an N95 mask does so that contaminants can get into the mask through those holes.

Similarly, cloth masks won't absorb the same amount of tiny particles as a surgical mask. N95 mask, one of the most powerful facial masks out there, just blocks 95 percent of small particles.

DON'T

1. Wear your mask only on the tip of your nose, or leave your nose exposed.

The virus spreads through breath droplets, which can penetrate through the nose and mouth. The mask will cover your face up to the bridge of your nose to ensure the nose is adequately covered. When too much is hidden by your nose, it can be a little stuffy, but wearing the mask under your nose makes it less effective.

2. Leave your chin exposed

Even like a mask is meant to cover the nose up to the nose bridge, so does a face mask protect the face under the chin. If your chin is left exposed to a mask, consider buying or making a larger one.

3. Leave spaces on the sides of the mask

A mask with facial gaps is quite ineffective in preventing the person wearing it from distributing breathable droplets. This also makes the blocking of droplets less effective for the mask. To ensure a snug fit, use the ear loops to secure the mask as much as possible.

4. Touch the mask or your face while using it

Once wearing, it can be easy to get the urge to brush your face or fidget with a face mask. You should also avoid touching your face to prevent the virus from spreading to your mouth, eyes, or nose. The outside of the mask is no longer clean when worn outdoors, so one can avoid touching it.

5. Pull the mask down under your jaw or off to the side while being used

You won't take off the veil/mask until you are back home and ready to discard or wash it. Try not to evacuate the veil and set it back on while you are out in the open, pull it down towards your jaw or slice one ear circle to hold it sideways. You can get stuffy when wearing a mask, removing it will reveal you prematurely.

6. Re-use single-use masks

Single-use masks should be used only once, such as those made from paper towels. Throw away such a face mask after you are done with it. For a new usage, use a new, clean, sterile mask.

7. Have a false sense of security

Wearing a mask will make you feel more comfortable than you are. Remembering to wear a mask isn't going to guarantee you won't catch the virus necessarily. The most effective way to defend yourself against COVID-19 is to stay home, wash your hands, and practice effective social distancing.

CHAPTER 6

THE RIGHT WAY TO USE AND CLEAN YOUR MASK

These handmade masks should cover your nose and ears, and they should be worn any time you're in a crowd, for example. B. In the Pharmacy or Store. A great deal of planning has been helpful for making a cover with the materials you'd have at home.

While N95 careful covers and respirators are supposed to be reserved for the essential personnel, the thought is that a basic wrap of material could keep asymptomatic individuals from spreading the malady in circumstances where social separation is hard to keep up.

"This is not to prevent you from becoming infected with viruses. It is to prevent other people from becoming infected by you." If everyone follows this suggestion carefully, the group will benefit. "But obtaining a mask is only part of the puzzle: it has to be used correctly for masks to be successful.

Focus On The Fit

The faces will fit snugly but still be comfortable, covering the entire nose and mouth and reaching under the chin. You should be able to breathe normally, but the mask's sides should fit around your nose.

In reality, wearing a mask can be irritating to a little bit. Wearers of eyeglasses may have difficulty with masks that have dark lenses, and breathing can be a little uncomfortable or congested. (Children two years and younger and people with breathing problems should not wear facial fabric covers.) If you feel limited or uncomfortable wearing a scarf over your face, make a mask.

Put It On Carefully

If you wear a home mask, bandana, headscarf, or surgical mask, one of the vital steps when putting on or removing a face cover is to use good hygiene especially of the hands, whether using a hand disinfectant or washing with detergent and water your hands.

Use the ear hooks to put the mask on your face such that it covers your mouth and nose very well such that you can easily breathe. If you have a nasal bridge in your mask, keep it close and place the headphones over your ears.

The same care should be taken to put on a headscarf, scarf, or fabric cover.

Should not contact the mask or cloth outside, which should become contaminated.

Do not touch the mask as you put it on. During your travel, you should not detach, change, or shift your mask.

Take It Off Carefully Too

A procedure exists in which a mask is removed. The trick is to avoid contaminating your hands inadvertently or to touch your face.

While evacuating the face cover, take specific consideration not to contact the front of the veil, eyes, nose, and mouth and wash your hands in the wake of taking care of the cover.

Realize that wearing a veil of texture or face covering doesn't make you powerful. You will get infectious particles from outside. Secure your protective equipment in a paper bag. Do the same with your fabric cover.

Clean the mask; sometimes, there are currently no strict protocols for cleaning and disinfecting facial garments and fabric masks.

It should be washed periodically, or after every use. The reuse of a fabric cover is perfect as long as it is not dirty.

Wait until the face cover is dirty to wash if you don't have immediate access to clothing. Any garments or accessories you wear could be tainted, but experts don't think the transmission process is so severe that you need to wash or change clothes multiple times a day, he says. For cloth masks and face linings, the same applies.

CHAPTER 7

DIY FACE MASKS TEMPLATE STEP BY STEP GUIDE

Utilize these free sewing examples and models to sew a face cover for DIY that you can give to an emergency clinic, specialist's office, social insurance laborers, or other principle workers. You can wash and re-utilize those veils. Many have channel packs that delay their lives.

You can sew one of these DIY face covers if you are good at sewing a straight line. It's a basic task that takes an exceptionally constrained measure of time to construct and needs just a couple of materials that you most likely as of now have. There are various structures and strategies to make them, yet all the accompanying plans structure a cover that can be worn by social insurance experts.

Filters And How Important They Are

Do you need a filter for your natively constructed face mask?

Specialists state adding a filter to confront masks may offer additional assurance to the wearer, rather than simply those close by.

Wearing a fabric face mask has become a standard piece of life when going out when there is some sort of pandemic. Face masks, which you can make from materials around the house, are intended to shield everyone around you from getting the infection. Research appears at half of individuals with COVID-19 don't show manifestations. However, in case you're hoping to give yourself additional security when out in the open, adding a filter to your natively constructed mask may work.

This is what you should think about face mask filters, should you choose to utilize one.

What do mask filters do?

In a perfect world, face mask filters will "improve the capacities of hand crafted, fabric masks.

A successful face mask filter will permit a ton of wind current while additionally catching a high level of the infection's particles.

What can you use when making a filter?

If, by chance, you can't obtain a HEPA filter, including more layers of a firmly woven texture can likewise support assurance. To check the viability of the texture, hold it up to the light. If you can notice its individual filaments, it's most likely not an incredible material.

You can tell if a filter won't permit sufficient wind stream by breathing through it while wearing glasses.

HEPA filters are significantly more viable.

How might you grimace mask with a filter?

Numerous masks accessible for buy online additionally accompany sewn pockets where you can include a filter. To crease the filter into your DIY mask, follow these means:

Face mask filter

Here is an instructional exercise on utilizing the filter:

Take a handkerchief or square bit of texture.

Crease the texture into equal parts.

Holding the material vertically, crease the top mostly down and the base most of the way up so they compromise.

Crease the base most of the way up once more.

Spot the filter on the top half and crease it down to the end.

Holding the material on a level plane, place elastic groups around the left and right parts of the bargains, leaving about an inch on either side.

Overlap the left and right finishes in toward the center so the elastic groups are on the very closures.

Spot the side with the collapsed closes against your nose and mouth.

Pull the elastic groups around your ears to hold set up.

In the event that you utilize a HEPA filter, you ought to consistently keep a layer of texture between the filter and your mouth. HEPA filters contain fiberglass, which you would prefer not to breathe in.

However, if you have a sewn mask without a pocket and need to utilize a HEPA filter, include another layer of texture between the filter and your face and ensure that you can inhale sufficiently. Significantly looser weave textures will extraordinarily decrease the danger of breathing in particles from the filter itself.

CHAPTER 8

FACTS ABOUT USING FACE MASKS

Since the start of the various virus outbreaks, many people have been advised not to use or wear face masks till they are ill or taking care of someone who is ill and unable to use one, or who works in health management or care.

This strategy is now undergoing major changes.

It is now recommended that people wear facial fabric covers in public places where other social isolation interventions are difficult to sustain to prevent the spread of viruses and other diseases.

There's a good reason for this change in approach: there's growing evidence that presymptomatic and asymptomatic carriers can spread the virus.

People are being told, however, not to wear medical masks, which are currently uncommon in hospitals. Which means one thing: just close is the age of DIY masks and face linings.

Can face coverings prevent the spread of the virus?

The biggest advantage of covering the face, mouth and nose is that it protects us. While there are still a lot to learn about viruses and other illnesses, it seems that people infected with one virus or another will infect others by coughing, sneezing, and other drops of breath.

For that reason, even though you don't feel weak or sick, it is still smart to wear a mask.

When you cough, sneeze or let out water while speaking, certain breath drops will be covered by the mask to prevent them from dropping on people or surfaces around. So it primarily shields your neighbor, not you. If your neighbor wears a mask and wants to do the same, they'll cover him. Therefore, properly fitted masks will help people." The N95 respirators are the best masks, but the public is advised not to use them since health workers are in desperate need of them at present. If you have them, you can donate them to a local hospital immediately. These slim blue versions, which provide less protection but are useful and uncommon, do the same to surgical masks.

If i'm wearing a mask and someone sneezes on me, would the mask offer some protection?

Yes, but if and only if you wear the mask the way it should be worn, and afterward do not let your lips touch it.

That is why masks struggle in studies: people don't rightly wear them. They hit the bands, and they make adjustments.

Somehow, they push it down to get out of their ears. "What that person coughed or sneezed is now in your hands if you touch the front of the mask. Another thing: Hopefully, you should also have eye protection to avoid the sneeze of a stranger from entering. Glasses and goggles are not ideal, but they can help.

What about homemade masks?

Some work has shown that the material on cotton T-shirts and tea towels can trap disease droplets, but the protection they provide is uncertain.

Another study of healthcare worker found that wearing fabric masks resulted in more infections than using surgical masks or a control group.

Yet people think it is a nice idea and have used one for their N95 masks. We also do not know exactly how powerful homemade masks are.

How often do i need to wash the face mask?

Think of a mask as underwear: after each use, it needs to be cleaned.

"You don't remove this filthy mask, put it inside your purse or pocket, and then put it again on your face. 'It's something that you can either cover your cough, sneeze, or spray your voice, or shield you from other people's coughs, spray, and expression. So it's filthy, now. This simply has to be either discarded or cleaned. "And if you wear a cloth mask, immediately place it in the laundry bin. If it's unused, throw it away. It's hugely wrong to remove the mask to eat or speak and the put it back on. You've already got the dirty stuff on your hands and through your mouth.

Individuals ought to be wearing fabric face covers to forestall the spread of infections and different pathogens

These hand crafted veils should cover the nose and mouth and be worn at whatever point you're in a network setting, such as heading off to the general store or drug store. The CDC has an accommodating aide for DIY-ing a veil with materials you'd have at home.

While careful covers and N95 respirators should be put something aside for human services laborers, the thought is that a basic fabric covering could keep asymptomatic individuals from dispersing the malady in circumstances where it's difficult to keep up social separation.

These are not expected to keep you from getting the infection, they are proposed to keep others from getting the infection from you. If everyone, no one excluded, takes that proposal cautiously, you are killing off the virus.

Yet, making sure about a veil is only one bit of the riddle: For covers to be powerful, they should be worn appropriately. Here's the correct method to utilize a material face covering during the COVID-19 pandemic, in addition to basic traps that could influence your security:

Concentrate on the fit

In truth, wearing a cover can be somewhat irritating. Glasses-wearers may battle with covers steaming up focal points, and it can make breathing to some degree awkward or stuffy. (Children under age 2 and individuals who experience difficulty breathing shouldn't wear fabric face covers, per the CDC.)

In case you're feeling limited or awkward wearing a scarf over your face, you might need to think about creation a cover. Here's the means by which the CDC recommends making a fast face covering utilizing a scarf, handkerchief or towel and two elastic groups or hair elastics.

Put it on cautiously

Even if you're utilizing a natively constructed veil, scarf, handkerchief or careful cover, one of the most vital strides before putting on or subsequent to removing a face covering is to utilize suitable hand cleanliness, either by utilizing hand sanitizer or washing properly your hands with soap and water.

The World Health Organization proposes that individuals first clean their hands before putting a cover on and watch that there are no gaps or tears in the texture.

When putting all over covering, utilize the connections to put it all over and spread your face and mouth cozily, ensuring you can inhale without any problem. In the event that your veil has a nose connect, hold it set up, at that point circle the ear groups over your ears.

A handkerchief, scarf or material covering ought to be applied with a similar consideration.

Also, don't contact the outside of the cover or material which could be polluted.

Try not to contact the cover while wearing it

You shouldn't be taking off, altering or moving your cover during your excursion.

It is imperative to recall the outside of the cover is viewed as sullied.

An ongoing lab study found that the infections could make due on a face cover for as long as seven days.

That implies, in the event that you should remove your veil for a snappy breather, or a tingle, it's imperative to rehearse great hand cleanliness in the wake of contacting the face covering.

Take it off cautiously as well

There's some method included removing a cover, particularly in case you're a human services laborer or dealing with somebody who has COVID-19. The key is to dodge unintentionally sullying your hands or contacting your face.

Be extra mindful so as not to touch the front of your veil and your eyes, mouth or nose while evacuating your face covering, and wash your hands subsequent to taking care of your veil, as indicated by the CDC.

As of now, there are no exacting rules about washing and sterilizing fabric face covers and veils. As indicated by the CDC, machine-washing your veil is sufficient to sanitize your fabric face covering.

Any dress or embellishments that you wear can possibly be defiled, yet right now specialists don't accept that the component of transmission is outrageous to such an extent that you should wash or putting on something else on various occasions a day, he says. The equivalent is valid for fabric veils and face covers.

Keep Your Social Distance

Wearing a face covering is only one extra advance that you can take to stop the spread of COVID-19, yet it is anything but a substitution for the other significant avoidance measures, for example, washing your hands and social removing.

Like different measures, it's critical to do your part. Anything that diminishes transmission right now has tremendous advantage to the general population.

Is there one best mask design?

So far, in general, there are few data on fabrics or home masks and far less data than decide how many folds you can put on your self-sewn version.

A tightly woven cotton is the very best material. "Don't use nylon or polyester because they have tested the survivability of the virus on fabrics, and the worst is spandex.

You can make a mask with a t-shirt, and you don't need a sewing machine. You can also try making one of them (unused) towels from the shop. But whatever you do, try to make it suit your face and don't touch your front until you've worn it out. If you are wearing cloth masks, make many so that each time you go out, you can wear one new.

Do masks confer any other benefits?

Masks can also act as an important visual indicator. We are a "reminder we need to take these steps and warn people to stay away to prevent unseen breaches." This will feel like an honor badge. Wearing a mask in public means I'm worried about you; I'm worried about my neighbors, I'm worried about strangers, I'm worried about getting poisoned. I want to do my part to minimize the effect this could have. It can also provide a sense of protection for the customer.

It seems like you're behind a sign, and I think that can be calming in itself. For the people around you, it's a message. At the moment, there's a health crisis; viruses are going on; we need to be vigilant.

How To Reduce Your Risk Of Infectious Diseases

There are some ways that have been proven to help keep yourself safe. You know the fundamental ones: stay away from dry cough and runny nose. You may wonder about other realistic ways to stay infection-free, though. That has become an even bigger problem. While vaccination and antibiotics have often minimized the risk associated with "traditional infections," new infectious diseases are new to remind us how fragile we are.

Not only do new "bugs" emerge, but even some of the "classic bugs" get cleverer. The skin serves as a natural barrier to toxic, infectious microbes. "Smart bugs" have, however, found new ways of entering the body and causing infections. Smart bugs have also evolved quickly to make links that can infect many of our existing antibiotic arsenals, and, in some cases, all of them. In an event that you've seen the updates on these developing infectious and savage maladies, you might be somewhat stressed. We as a whole appear to know somebody who was basically sound yet who obtained a type of infection that caused genuine disease and inability. Is it likely you could be next time?

While the sharpest individual can be frightened by both old and new pathogens, we are not without measures to battle them. You can without much of a stretch forestall the spread of numerous irresistible infections by making a couple of simple conduct changes (which at long last will lessen your body get to).

We should take a gander at ten practical tips for diminishing the hazard, trailed by some particular guidance for the individuals who are pregnant or immunosuppressed because of sickness or chemo. A portion of these tips may sound straightforward; others may stun you.

Wash Your Hands Frequently And Well

Do you realize microorganisms can live on idle surfaces from two or three minutes to months?

It depends on microorganism and the earth. Some can live just for a short time; others will live long. Envision these illness causing microorganisms which live close to the crosswalk on your PC console, your light switch, or even the crosswalk button! Fomites can transmit numerous diseases. This word characterizes the arbiter that is among you and someone else contaminated.

Most by far of individuals don't have the foggiest idea how to wash their appearances appropriately. It is prescribed to wash completely and overwhelmingly for in any event 20 seconds with water and cleanser and afterward dry by hand or with a spotless towel in the sun.

A liquor based gel or a hand wash is proper without running water, yet nothing is superior to plain old cleanser and water. This takes nearly insofar as singing a song like "Happy Birthday," which is the reason a few emergency clinics suggest that you wash your hands for this simple melody to last!

Try not to SHARE PERSONAL ITEMS

Irresistible specialists (microorganisms, infections, and parasites) may incorporate toothbrushes, towels, razors, cloths, and nail scissors. They told you in kindergarten the best way to share your toys, yet they hushed up about their hands. Presently, make sure to keep your own assets! For instance, sharing razors and toothbrushes can transmit hepatitis.

Spread YOUR MOUTH WHEN YOU COUGH OR SNEEZE

Similarly, great individual cleanliness requires individual neatness as well as the hundreds of years old convention of hacking or sniffling up your mouth. For what reason is this essential when you don't feel wiped out? The sickness causing microorganism has just started to develop with most contaminations and to separate some time before indications show up.

These germs can be transmitted by infinitesimal beads noticeable all around by hacking or sniffling. The present suggestion is that as opposed to utilizing your exposed hands, you spread your mouth with your neck, sleeve, or elbow.

Get Vaccinated

It's said the resistant framework has a "memory" of past contaminations. In the event that your body distinguishes an organism that has just set off a contamination, this will expand the improvement of white platelets and antibodies a subsequent time to keep away from disease. On the off chance that you get immunized, in any case, you "imagine" that your body has been undermined by a particular microorganism, accordingly fortifying its insurance against resulting diseases.

At the point when you get the immunizations you need, you're protected, alongside your environment. For instance, hepatitis B inoculation is a methods for ensuring yourself, regardless of whether it isn't sufficient to utilize the individual things of others.

Utilize Safe Cooking Practices

Stomach related sicknesses are frequently the consequence of lack of foresight and dietary patterns. What a few people neglect to know is that most of grown-up instances of "stomach influenza" are likely food contamination. Organisms prosper in practically all nourishments, and all the more so in nourishments that are kept at room temperature.

Chilling eases back off or forestalls the advancement of most microorganisms. Promptly set the nourishment into the refrigerator inside two hours of readiness. In case you're thinking about what to do together at your next dinner, look at those sanitation tips while barbecuing and picnicking. For crude meat and vegetables, utilize distinctive cutting sheets, keep your ledges clean and wash all the foods grown from the ground a long time before eating.

Be A Smart Traveler

Irresistible infections can be effectively recognized while voyaging, particularly on the off chance that you travel to asset constrained nations. On the off chance that your movement goal is where water is rare, ensure that a decent wellspring of water, for example, mineral water, is utilized to drink and brush your teeth. Recollect that occasionally ice solid shapes can be a "covered up" wellspring of debased water.

Eat prepared nourishment, and dodge crude vegetables and natural products. Pick those that can be stripped when eating organic product, and ensure the strip doesn't come into contact with the remainder of the natural product when stripping. At long last, update your movement goal with any fundamental or required inoculations.

Practice Safe Sex

Explicitly transmitted illnesses are maybe the most effectively preventable of irresistible ailments. Managing safe sex (with condoms) may forestall irresistible microscopic organisms or infections from spreading starting with one individual then onto the next.

Not simply irresistible ailment or even pregnancy can be an issue. It is evaluated that around 16 percent of malignancies overall are related with diseases, a large portion of which are transmitted explicitly.

Try Not to Pick Your Nose (Or Your Mouth and Eyes)

In addition to the fact that it is a social forbidden, yet the pricking of the nose permits an assortment of sicknesses to spread. Glance around and perceive what number of individuals have their hands over their mouths. Numerous microorganisms lean toward the dry, wet nose atmosphere, just as different surfaces secured with bodily fluid, for example, the eyes and mouth. By not entering certain spots, diseases can be effectively maintained a strategic distance from.

Exercise Caution with Animals

Contaminations that can be spread from creatures to people are viewed as zoonotic ailments, and they are more typical than a great many people accept. On the off chance that you have pets, make sure that you have every day tests and that the immunizations are exceptional. Every now and again clean the litter boxes (except if you're pregnant, remain away!) and protect little children from creature droppings.

Various types of untamed life can transmit ailments, for example, rabies or avian flu, and plague and Lyme ailment can spread bugs and ticks. Make the earth around your home risky to rodents and different warm blooded creatures by maintaining a strategic distance from places where they can stow away or manufacture nooks, utilizing disposed of rat safe waste jars and bolting openings that make it advantageous and enticing for creatures to enter. Encourage small kids to be wary when they go over wild creatures in your neighborhood.

Watch The News

A decent comprehension of recent developments can assist you with settling on savvy travel or other recreation choices. A flying creature influenza episode in Asia, for instance, may make you reconsider before arranging an outing. Holes of mosquito-spreading West Nile infection? Maybe on your outdoors trip, you need to bring bug shower! In Peppers, Salmonella? Try not to benefit from tomatoes. You get the image. The CDC offers online data about the latest flare-ups and the world's zones where numerous irresistible infections are common.

For Those Who Are Pregnant

The individuals who are pregnant need extra checking. A few contaminations that solitary trouble solid individuals who are not pregnant, during pregnancy can cause issues. Numerous illnesses can prompt unnatural birth cycles and stillbirths, while others can prompt inherent handicaps.

You ought not consider pregnancy. The intercessions referenced above on contamination avoidance are compelling in lessening your hazard.

For Those in The Hospital

Medical clinic gained diseases, known as "nosocomial contaminations," are a noteworthy reason for death in certain locales. Notwithstanding being a touch of rearing ground for awful microscopic organisms, the emergency clinic has likewise settled protection from a considerable lot of these microorganisms. Most anti-infection agents.

For Those Who Are Immunosuppressed or On Chemotherapy

For those experiencing chemotherapy, HIV-tainted, or immunosuppressed, shielding themselves from tiny dangers requires more vitality. Microscopic organisms that don't cause contaminations can turn into an issue in individuals with a sound invulnerable framework (artful diseases) and these individuals can likewise turn out to be a lot more wiped out when presented to contaminations.

Counting pet-borne contaminations to nourishment borne diseases, you ought to gain proficiency with a couple of things about contaminations that go past the above anticipation tips. Expertise to diminish your danger of contamination during chemotherapy, or if for some other reason, your safe framework is undermined.

Disclaimer

This book is not meant as a replacement for the medical advice from doctors and other medical personnel physicians.

The reader should regularly consult a physician in matters relating to his/her health and particularly with respect to any symptoms that may require diagnosis or medical attention.

Do Not Go Yet; One Last Thing To Do

If you enjoyed this book or found it useful, I'd be very grateful if you'd post a short review on Amazon. Your support does make a difference, and I read all the reviews personally so I can get your feedback and make this book even better.

Thanks again for your support!